Contents

Introduction

Hi. As young adults, the daunting thought of having to avoid foods or make restrictions horrifies us and ill health seems so far from the now. I'm here to tell you that health problems will happen if you act careless and treat your health likes it's too far away to be a concern. Honestly it's not that far at all. What my diligent colleagues and I hope you take away from this book is not only should you be concerned now, but how aware and involved you need to be.

 As true with literally anything else, as you practice the healthy lifestyle choices in this book they will become more second nature to you and soon enough, you won't realize that you're alive for longer than others. It sounds depressing but this stuff is pretty important. Hopefully we can teach you how important it is to live healthy and have fun.

 Keep in mind that this book is only really designed to give you a brief glimpse into the vast world of public health. Public health is the often-untouched area of medicine that's arguably the most important part.

Public health departments are responsible for 5 main areas, epidemiology, biotechnology, social behavioral and community health, environmental health, and public policy. Each of these sections deserve a 500 page book or 2 but I'm not that good at writing so I'll just briefly explain what each area is about.

First you have epidemiology. This is the biggest division and one of the most important divisions in public health. Epidemiologists are the people that do all the research you see in medicine and general studies. There are multiple types of epidemiologists and they each have different roles but I'm not going to bore you with the nitty gritty details.

Next you have biotechnology which is another important section but I have a feeling I'm gonna be saying that about every section. They are responsible for developing technology that extends the duration of a humans life at all costs. This honorable division helps improve wheelchairs, portable oxygen tanks and now even bionic limbs.

Third you have social behavioral and community health department. This department handles the outreach part of public health. What good is finding the cure to AIDS and not making it available to the public? They build clinics that offer emergency services and make vaccines easily accessible to all. It is the division that encompasses this book.

Then you have environmental health. These guys are the ones responsible for pushing for a cleaner earth. They study the effects humans have on Earth and they discover how to prevent the end of the world. While what they do is great, it's also great if people listen to them *wink* *wink*.

Last but not least is public policy. These guys have the job of passing laws that preserve life and follow the research their public health pals record. They release the laws and regulations that limit carbon monoxide emitted, require seatbelt use, put fluoride in water, and many other things that would help keep the earth spinning and you living healthy in it.

Though they seem different, all 5 of these divisions are centered on one main focus, that focus being educating humans in health literacy. Health literacy and health education are actually different. Health education is kind of the guidelines and steps on how to lead a healthy life. Health literacy is more about how the health "code" applies to your own life. This can be interpreted in 2 different ways, education is what your body needs to stay healthy and health literacy is how you adapt it to your own lifestyle. I'll tell you right now that you aren't gonna stick with your healthy style changes if they compete with your traditional day.

I can't tell you a really effective way of applying these health tips because it's your life, but some helpful tips on how to integrate a healthy lifestyle are substitution, replacement and abolishment. Basically substitute unhealthy choices for healthy ones, preferably so that you barely notice the change. Replace unhealthy parts with parts that are better for you. This could be food, people or activities. Finally, you have to totally get rid of some things that are just plain stupid. Stuff like recreational drugs and alcohol have no substitute and should be stopped immediately. We will discuss drugs later. For now the biggest tip to properly applying health literacy to your life is to know stuff.

What the Heck is Health?

That question probably sounds pretty stupid huh? I felt kinda stupid typing it. Quite frankly, that's a question a lot of people have a hard time answering. Probably too many people. Health, if you haven't figured out by now, is very important to each and every human on earth. Believe it or not, it isn't just eating vegetables and not eating junk food. Health, in its basics, can be broken into 4 sections; physical, mental, social and spiritual.

First is physical, and this branch of health is massive. Physical health doesn't necessarily mean bench pressing 300 pounds or running a marathon. It can simply consist of taking your dog on a walk today or walking to school. Physical health basically means using the calories you gain throughout the day. Do this and you won't be at risk of obesity or other physical ailments. Physical health is just what you can do with your body. Food, exercise, sleep, and drinking water helps you do it better.

The next branch of health is mental health. This is as simple as having a brighter outlook on life and as complicated as having plaques form on your brain causing the erasing of your life's memories. Though mental health is something we still don't fully understand, there are step to take that prevent mental breakdowns. Being healthy with what you eat is vital to keeping a healthy mind but sometimes you can't help it because of events you experience. Event-caused mental illnesses often consist of PTSD, paranoia and others. Mental health problems most frequently are diagnosed between 16 and 24. If you don't feel like the same person you were, consider talking to someone.

The Third branch is social health. Another way to lessen the risk of mental illness is by being more socially involved. Though it seems silly and stupid, there is a metric ton of scientific studies done on various effects of proper social health and what it looks like without it. The thing with social health is that it can lead to some detrimental effects if you don't have it, but having it simply means being around people and talking to people. Each person has a different "gauge" to determine how much you could need, but the key is finding yours.

Finally is spiritual health. This ironically also relates to physical, mental and social health, as your choice of religious belief holds a great impact on your lifestyle and choices. Choosing to believe in a religion often has more benefits for you that are incorporated and also gives one a sense of hope and aspiration, something a non-religious person would be slightly more hard-pressed to find. It is all a personal preference but the key is to be at peace with what you stand for and represent, because not being so has a lot of negative effects.

How to Manage Your Medical Care and Tips on Finding the Right Doctor

Having a doctor you trust is critical because you will be more open and forthcoming to your doctor about issues you may be facing. This is the same with insurance and medical care. In this section we will be discussing how to approach getting a doctor, especially a new one. We will also cover on how to interpret medical info you might receive.

Getting a new doctor can be a scary task, but it's a skill everyone uses at least once their life. The main key is to "write out your story". Now whether this means actually writing it out or just sitting down and thinking through what you have to say, it's always helpful to compile your medical history before you go to your doctor rather than thinking of it off the spot. Your medical history can be nailed down by what medications you've had to take. Having a headache is very different from having chronic migraines. Ignore most of the common sicknesses, address only the big diseases or conditions you have had in the past or that you may currently have. Though it may seem unimportant, the order in which you got sick may be helpful to your new doctor, but it isn't critical so don't sweat if you can't remember if you got mono before or after your measles infection.

In order to construct your "story" you may have to reference some old medical documents. Before anything else, just make sure you KEEP EVERY

MEDICAL DOCUMENT IN A SORTED AREA!!! I cannot stress the importance of this enough. No matter how pointless or useless a document or receipt you receive may look, keep it. You never know when you may be asked to reference something and it will be a lot simpler if you have the document ready to present.

You also need to be able to read and understand those forms. This is something that really shouldn't need to be covered especially because you can obviously read if you're reading this, but believe it or not, some people still don't know how. If that's the case, you will need to have someone show you how to read your medical documents. As long as you sort and keep all your medical documents then you will be good to go.

You need to be able to have a comfortable conversation with your doctor. If you can't, you need to find a new one. Don't stay with a doctor who doesn't understand your values, is dismissive of your concerns, or makes you feel queasy at the thought of sharing your decisions with. You may have to suck it up and deal with a bad teacher, but you never have to deal with a bad doctor. Fire them immediately and find a new one you like. Ask your insurance provider, your Facebook friends, or your family who they like.

Communicating with your health care professional and drug advice

Your doctor is trying to keep you alive. The tricky thing is that he/she isn't constantly observing our life from a TV in their living room. What this means is that in order for your doctor to successfully keep you living, you need to communicate with them.

First, you need to schedule an appointment. This step is pretty scary to some people but you will soon learn the secretary you reach is very helpful and only wants to make life easy for everyone. Simply indicate why you want to make an appointment and tell them when you are available.

Next is at the office. As discussed in the last section, be sure to bring any medical documents you have. For a usual check-up the nurse will check your weight, blood pressure, eyes and ears, and your height. If the nurse asks any questions, answer them to the best of your ability, but usually this step can be done pretty quietly.

After receiving your check-in screening by the nurse, the doctor should meet with you. The doctor should ask you why you scheduled an appointment. This part is when you describe the symptoms you felt that encouraged you to see the doctor. ANSWER WITH COMPLETE HONESTY!!! Don't blow things out of proportion because this can cause misdiagnoses which are annoying, expensive and sometimes deadly. The doctor may ask for a blood or urine sample. Keep in mind not all doctor visits may go this way. Be open minded and ready to answer any questions, and remember that doctors aren't heartless and are always trying to help. An easy way to ensure you heard correctly all the info provided is the teach-back method. Simply repeat the info you heard to your doctor and they should correct you and stress any important details you may have missed.

The other important part of communication is with medication. Medication is obviously very important and very easy to make mistakes with. Though sometimes a dose or medication mistake can be harmless, other time it can be very deadly. If you properly describe your symptoms to your doctor and your doctor properly understands and diagnoses you, you really won't have much to worry about other than making sure you take the correct amount of pills. I don't care if you think your doctor is stupid or that he miss-diagnosed you, listen to your doctor. If something ends up being wrong, your doctor will be fully responsible.

As someone taking a medication, you must also be aware of other medicines you may be taking. Occasionally, medicines counteract against each other and cause nasty symptoms you would be better off avoiding. Though this is rare, make sure that you communicate to your doctor about medications you are currently taking or have taken in the past.

Medications are more than what your doctor prescribes you that you must go to a pharmacist for. Medications are anything you put in or on your body to make you feel better or to improve your health. That includes over the counter drugs, vitamins, minerals, herbal supplements, and weird nutritional shakes your coach or mother makes you drink. It also includes alcohol and illegal drugs. Make sure all medications you take are in your medical records and part of your health story.

How Healthy Life Choices Will Make You Healthy. Duh!

Most people know what healthy choices are, but we are going to discuss this along with what you might need to change.

Healthy food choices can be made by simply applying one rule; don't eat stuff you can't pronounce. Almost all harmful food ingredients and products that have confusing names are harmful and should be avoided. You can also use price clues, because unhealthy foods usually tend to be cheaper than their more healthy brothers. You also want to incorporate less sugars and more fruits and vegetables. Ugh right?

One of the fun parts about health literacy is actually learning to cook and substituting unhealthy choices for healthy ones. This could mean making your own chips, creating a healthy flavorful drink, and more. Aiming to eat 5 to 7 fruit and vegetables a day and cutting salt and fat are really the two best rules. If you use these simple steps, implementing a healthy diet will be a breeze.

Also you want to drink tons of water. Water does a lot of great things for humans (alongside keeping us alive) that really benefit to have. It's usually best if men drink 13 glasses of water, and women 9 glasses a day, but keep in mind beverages like coffee and juice can be include that water content.

Healthy activities are another great way to stay physically and mentally healthy.

Learning to reduce your stress is key to living healthy. Meditation is great ways to leave your mind healthy and mentally stable. Meditation has been in a ton of studies that reveal just taking 10 minutes to seal out everything happening around you can drastically increase productivity. Getting fresh air, a massage, swinging, singing loudly, and playing games all help us relax. When you stumble on something that helps you to calm down, do it. Often.

Sleep is also key in operating properly. Getting at least 8 hours of sleep a day will do the job perfectly but sometimes you need to catch up on sleep with an hour long nap. Do yourself a huge favor and don't deny you're body the sleep that it needs. You will barely function without sleep and stuff like energy drinks won't help. When you sleep, your body heals itself and your brain processes information from short-term to long-term memory. That means sleeping is a form of studying!

Exercise is something that is really good for people who want it, but lots of people say they don't have time for it.

There have also been a number of studies done showing the numerous mental benefits of exercise, especially running. Hundreds of studies showing that running is the best thing you can do to boost your mind. If this isn't your favorite thing to do though, anything else you do is also somehow helpful. Just getting your blood moving and walking to Walmart or the nearest corner store helps. Move more in all the simple ways.

If you take a couple minutes to do something that can improve your whole life it will be a really good thing for you and your body. Even a few minutes out of your day for exercise will help you understand what it does for your body and how good it is for your health.

A personal story from Qudratullah

Not everyone likes to eat vegetables, but you really need to eat heathy foods because if you start working out and not eating right, your weight will grow and you will not get the health benefits of exercise.

It's healthy to exercise a couple times a week. That includes exercises like running and other sports that you can play. If you regularly play sports you don't need to do other exercise because playing any sport is good exercise.

A lot of Americans don't exercise because they don't like it or they don't have time for it. If you start to exercise from a young age, by the time you grow up you will have really good health habits and really good life.

I'm always trying new sports. When I first came to United States I was really weak, so I started going to boxing. In 7th grade, I started wrestling. My coach is a great man who helped us a lot with practice for a match and for other kind of things to help us to make good choices about what to eat and what to not eat.

The reason team sports are so good for you is that they boost your social health.

You learn good habits from your coach, and you make lots of friends who can be like family.

My favorite sport is cricket. I like it because my dad taught me how to play before he died and because it is really fun.

What is cricket? Cricket is a little bit like baseball. On each team we have 12 people who are play as ballers and batters.

Almost every country except America has a national team. My whole family plays cricket. My goal is to start an American cricket team.

Anyone can get a lot of exercise on a cricket team. Every year cricket has a world cup, similar to soccer. This year England won the world cup in overtime.

I am always trying to be what my family wants me to be and be the most famous cricket player in the world.

That way I can be a role model for good health and exercise. Maybe people will see me and wonder how I stay in shape and want to be like me. Maybe they'll learn how to play cricket or another team sport. Maybe they will start to exercise and see the change in their own bodies, too.

You don't have to be rich or go to a fancy gym to be healthy for your whole life. You can play sports your whole life, with a team or with your family. Do this and you will live longer and be happier.

Smoking

Just don't. No one thinks it's cool, no one wants to smell them and no one likes what it does to people. The advertisements that share the symptoms and complications of using cigarettes are completely true. Here are just a miniscule amount of the things that could happen to you.

1. You are more likely to get all forms of cancer than non-smokers

2. Non-smokers too can get cancer by breathing in the smoke that a smoker releases in the air

3. You can get Buerger's Disease, which swells blood vessels and prevents blood flow in your arms and legs. This can lead to pain, tissue damage and gangrene (death of body tissues). An amputation may or may not be required.

4. Increased risk of heart failure

5. If you have asthma, you can have an asthma attack thanks to the cigarette smoke others breathe.

6. If you have HIV and you smoke, you're more likely to get HIV infections including thrushes (mouth infection), Hairy leukoplakia (white mouth sores), bacterial pneumonia, and pneumocystis pneumonia, a dangerous lung infection

If you or someone you know smokes, you may need an emotional boost to quit for good. This website provides many inspiring stories of former smokers and how they learned to quit.

https://www.cdc.gov/tobacco/campaign/ 10Ya64wIVzICfCh3_TAcJEAAYASAAE glgZPD_BwE&gclsrc=aw.ds

Vaping is just as dangerous as a cigarette and causes a colorful variety of diseases and conditions no human should experience. Listed below are a couple of the bad things about vaping.

1. Vapes (particularly JUUL Co.) has more nicotine than a pack of 20 cigarettes

2. Stunts development of human brain

3. Causes a stronger addiction than cigarettes

4. You can lose your ability to focus properly

5. The e-cigarette has been known to explode, causing severe injury

6. Teens have been poisoned by breathing, swallowing or absorbing e-cigarette liquid through their eyes

7. E-cigarette aerosol isn't harmless water vapor

8. Most e-cigarettes on the market lie when they say they don't contain nicotine

Don't do anything here, please. I'm trying to live in a world with clean air and healthy people that are alive. I can't do it alone, so we need to all commit to not smoking or vaping.

Alcohol

Alcoholism is an issue that rips families apart and leaves relationships in tatters.

Listed below are some causes that may lead to someone becoming an alcoholic.

1. Family History. If your family has a history of alcohol abuse, you're more likely to become an alcoholic yourself

2. People who experienced a traumatic event of any sort are more likely to be an alcoholic

3. Poor family supervision also puts you at risk.

4. Peer pressure: societal pressure and influences, such as being given the impression through the media that alcohol use is a normal way to deal with stress can also increase the risk for individuals to abuse alcohol

5. The earlier you start to drink, the more likely you'll continue to do so.

Alcohol and drugs are often experimented with at our age. But when you do it alone or find you are having arguments with families and friends about your behavior, it's time to seek professional help.

College: Growing Up Quickly

College is a key example of where you will exercise the healthy living techniques you create for yourself, and this is due to a couple things. First off, your parents aren't responsible for you anymore. Medically when you turn 18, you are an adult. And as a student on a college campus, even if you are under 18, your parents are not allowed to know about how you are doing, unless you sign waivers allowing them to know some things. Whether you still live with your family, but you have your own bedtime or you live in a whole separate country, college is about being independent. You have to manage medical info, financial info, and taxes all by yourself. This seems pretty daunting cause it is. If you jack up money stuff you could very well end up on the streets. I have good news though. You can get by using a couple helpful steps. Don't waste your money on useless stuff, save, work, stay healthy, study and you should pass juuuuust fine.

It's important that while you manage your life you also manage your body, and this seems annoying and not entirely necessary. It doesn't have to be annoying, and it is very necessary. Simply fit a 1 mile jog in before heading to biochemistry or spend 45 minutes at the gym. The reason this may seem annoying is that you have things you would prefer to do over working out and I completely get it. The key is to not look at it as an annoying thing, but as a privilege that you can even do it. Say to yourself that you can so you should cause it will end up hurting you if you don't. Search until you find something you like doing. Some people actually enjoy exercise. I don't get you.

College is a real easy way to become a mindless addict to alcohol, drugs, sex and food. It is so important that you don't start unhealthy habits that are hard to break later.

Many college students get addicted to caffeine. The desire to stay up late and the need to get up early, may slow you down to the point where you depend on energy drinks to stay awake. Every once in a while, it's definitely ok, but every day use and you will buy a one- way ticket to the emergency room. Just ask my uncle.

Instead, substitute hundreds of dollars in monsters with sleep. Adults need 7-8 hours of sleep per night and teens who are studying may need 8-9. It's easy, goes by fast and is absolutely free! You will not only find yourself awake during lectures but you will retain the info and you won't feel like utter garbage all the time. It's really important that you manage your college life well because college is expensive and you do not want to waste all that money.

Colleges are also a unique area for seeking healthcare. All college campus' have mental health care, counseling centers, and assistance for those with any kind of disability right on the campus.

For physical health needs, you may have a college infirmary on the campus, or just off the campus. Community Colleges and smaller 4-year schools may not have medical offices onsite and you may need to use a local urgent care or emergency room if you are sick or injured. Make sure you know where to find mental and physical health help. You may not need it, but I can guarantee you will meet someone who does. And while you are at it, consider taking a first aid and CPR class so that you know what to do in an emergency.

Drugs, the Gateway into Homelessness, Bankruptcy and a Horribly Unhealthy Life

Yes that excessively long made the draft, but I think it properly captures a portion of what drug addiction can do to you and everyone around you. You can truly ruin yourself and your loved ones in tons of ways. The important thing to ask is "all for what?" and "is this worth it?" Obviously, it isn't, but maybe asking the question out loud will help you get a view of what you're doing. Before we continue, weed or marijuana is a drug and slowly our country is getting used to the concept that it has excellent medical uses. You wouldn't take your grandfather's high blood pressure medication, don't use marijuana either unless you are treating an illness you have. Pot is highly effective on seizures, anxiety, post traumatic stress disorders, and appetite issues.

First up is codeine. Codeine is regularly given because it's a common painkiller used to treat big and small problems including common colds. It's when people start chugging bottles of it that the problems arise. Codeine, often referred to as lean when mixed with its partner in crime, Sprite, leaves the abuser with slurred speech, anti-sociality and deep cravings that lead to the forgery of medical documents and stealing it from others. Lean doesn't cause many psychiatric effects to an abuser other than drastic mood swings. This is the least lethal drug but it is also the one that could most affect you due to its level of accessibility and ease to obtain. Keep in mind that it also can lead to hospitalization.

Next up on the roster of life ruining choices is crack. Professionally referred to as cocaine, this white powder you inhale through your nose is notorious for causing users to be hyperactive, socially awkward and isolated from others. You can usually tell when someone is high if their pupils are dilated and they lose excessive weight. They look like walking skeletons. High people tend to be stranger and crazier than usual. Also keep an eye out for white residue around their nose. Though crack is probably the second least lethal drug here, that doesn't mean its ok. You can still overdose and while you're high you can harm others and yourself and you wouldn't know it.

Third is heroin. This drug is horrible. It must be injected by needles or it can be snorted when held over an open flame, often times on a spoon.

The symptoms include depression, euphoria, mood swings, anxiety, hostility toward others, agitation and irritability, Lying about drug use, avoiding loved ones, weight loss, scabs or bruises as the result of picking at the skin, delusions, disorientation, hallucinations, paranoia, decreased attention to personal hygiene are all symptoms caused by continued use.

Possession of burned spoons, needles or syringes, missing shoelaces, glass pipes may be evidence of use. Stashing drug in various places around the home, car, and work, periods of hyperactivity followed by periods of exhaustion, inability to fulfill responsibilities at work or school, increased sleeping, apathy and lack of motivation, decline in occupational or academic performance can wreak havoc on college or careers.

Slurred speech, shortness of breath, frequent respiratory infections, dry mouth, wearing long pants and shirts, even in warm weather are additional symptoms. Going "on the nod" during conversations, walking zombie-like, forced, speech, track marks on arms and legs, warm, flushed skin, constricted pupils, and extreme itching are additional signs that someone is using.

That is a whole page of known heroin symptoms. You are also highly susceptible to overdosing, which is often fatal. This drug is often considered the extreme of drug usage. DON'T. DO. IT. If you want to live you will stay as far away from this drug as possible.

Finally is crystal meth or methamphetamine. This drug is the second worst here, due to the social changes it inflicts upon a user. Abusers experience loss of interest in usual activities, neglect relationships, isolate themselves from others, or have a sudden shift in social groups.

Risky financial behavior, such as cashing out savings in order to buy meth, criminality, such as stealing money or robbing stores are common. Obsessive focus on a particular issue or tasks, forgetting important dates, times or events, increased aggression or violent behavior, clumsiness can all follow use of this drug. Distracted behavior in social situations, risky sexual behavior, erratic sleep patterns (not sleeping or sleeping for more than 12 hours in a stretch), hyperactivity and high energy make keeping friends more difficult. Extreme loss of appetite (eating little or not at all for several days), and displaying a tic or twitch (a small, repetitive behavior, such as pulling hair or picking at a particular spot on the skin) are additional problem behaviors that sometimes never go away. This drug is more impactful socially than any other. It is also usually fatal if a user overdoses.

Some people may try to experiment with pills- oxycodone, Adderall, antidepressants and other meds are often handed out at parties along with alcohol. Don't try them. You have no idea what they are, how they will impact your body, or what other chemicals have been added to the drugs that could make you ill or kill you.

The drugs listed here are just a few of the many ways you can get high. Also, not listed here are withdrawal effects, some of which are worse than use effects. (People sobering up from alcohol can die in the withdrawal process.) Overall, drug use is something that ruins you and honestly isn't worth it. If you or anyone you know are stuck on drugs, call **(855) 311-7031** now.

Depression and Suicide

A lot of what this book has been about is partially keeping your body alive, but some of it actually is to keep you from depression. Depression is what eventually leads to suicide. Clinical depression is often due more to your brain chemistry and hormones. This could have been there at birth or appear during your life, often in your teen years. It may be genetic- your family members also have depression. Whatever the case, there is usually an outside trigger for your depression.

Depression can also be caused by trauma. Child abuse, unstable housing, assaults, and bullying can all trigger your brain to feel unsafe and overwhelmed by life and that can cause depression or anxiety.

DEPRESSION DOES NOT MEAN BEING SAD. Sadness is a momentary emotion one experiences in reaction to bad life moments. Depression tends to be a more unenergetic long-term sadness that is difficult to explain. What that basically means is that you shouldn't be sad but you are and you have no clue why.

Depression really sucks. Like really badly. Whether you have it or anyone you know has it, we can all agree that it is absolutely horrible. As people on the sidelines, it is our duty to make sure anyone who might be depressed knows we are here.

These 10 signs of depression should help. If you recognize yourself or a friend in this, please get help.

1. Consistent sadness, anxiety (low-grade fear)

2. Hopelessness, emptiness

3. Feelings of guilt and worthlessness

4. Lack of interest in things you enjoy

5. Constantly feeling tired, or exhausted

6. Inability to concentrate or focus

7. Sleep problems: insomnia, waking up very early, or waking up very late

8. Eating too much or not eating enough

9. Being restless or constantly irritated

10. Having suicidal thoughts or even attempting it.

There are many things you can do to treat depression. You could call the National Suicide Prevention Hotline at **1-800-273-8255** at any time. They are available 24/7. You could do is seek out counseling. The website **www.betterhelp.com/counselors** has over 1,500 trained counselors with at least 3 years and 2,000 hours of hands-on experience. Not every counselor you meet up with you will like. But, whatever you do, do not give up.

A Personal Story

The following story was bravely submitted by Brandon Cataldo

When I was in elementary school, I was constantly bullied for a wide range of reasons. The main ones were having autism and ADHD and because I never wore the popular clothes. My biggest regret was talking to the wrong people about it. I constantly told people who were not trustworthy. The teachers I told did nothing to help.

Another regret I have was not properly bringing it to my mother's attention of how all the bullying was affecting me. I never told my mother because I didn't want her to know I was struggling. I didn't want her to think I was a failure. Because I never told her, I started hating school. In 8th grade, I was at my lowest point. I wasn't suicidal, but I wasn't doing well mentally. I absolutely hated myself.

Despite the constant bullying, I managed to have 2 amazing friendships in my old school district before changing districts in 9th grade. Other than them, I had no friends. It was lonely, until I entered drama class on my first day. That day, I met a bunch of nice people who respected me for being myself rather than living up to conformity. Over time, I made lots of friends and as a result, I stopped hating myself. Now, despite not telling anyone helpful about my struggles, I turned out fine. I got lucky. Take it from me. Talk to someone you trust if you're struggling with your mental health. Not everyone is going to be as lucky as I was.

Keeping Your Pants Dry During the Apocalypse

Despite living in a gleaming, buttery society where your personal health is a main concern, things still happen. There are several community situations you have to be aware of, some human caused, some natural. In this section we will discuss how you deal with them because you definitely will know of them.

Boil Water

First is boil water advisories. You have probably never heard of this and honestly neither did I, but basically whenever a plumbing or water issue occurs on a massive scale, your city or town will issue a boil water advisory.

This means often times that a large water main has broken, but other times can mean a sewage floods are overwhelming water treatment efforts. If this is the case, you must boil all water you use, including drinking water, cooking water, hygienic water and pet drinking water. You must bring the water to a full rolling boil with lots of large bubbles for a minute and then cool the water back to room temperature, before it is safe to use.

Some uses of water already heat the water (clothes washing, dish washing) so that isn't a concern but be wary of shower water as it can still contain bacteria. If a water main is broken, you won't be able to use water summoning devices in your house at all. This means no tap water. Seeing as water is just a bit vital to human survival, you will have to buy water from your local grocery store, but other than that a broken water main will not impact you much. Your city will soon repair it and everything will be back to normal.

Food Recalls

Next is food recalls. Now this doesn't sound too apocalyptic, but if you're not careful you could start an outbreak. Food recalls will occur when a food retailer or manufacturer realizes that a product released and sold may have traces of a disease or bacteria. This could be due to equipment malfunction, but it is usually due to various other causes. If a food recall is issued, you will usually see it on multiple news networks, then you simply have to return it to the store you purchased it from. No receipt is usually required and you should be fully reimbursed for your purchase. Food recalls also occur when a potentially dangerous labeling mistake has been detected. This frequently happens, but usually is caught before it reaches the store. If the food does reach the store, it usually means a product has been printed with false allergy info or none at all. Simply return it if you have allergies and if not then you are going to be fine.

Food recalls are most dangerous to people who have health concerns already, especially the elderly, young children and diabetics.

Power

We all depend on electricity a lot. This means you need to be prepared for it to be snatched away from you. A brief power outage can range from a couple minutes to an half hour. These are never a concern, unless you depend on electrical medical technology to survive, in which you should always have a spare generator on stand-by.

Power outages of longer duration, however, can be a bit worse. The main risk is that all your refrigeration and lighting will be offline, risking that all your food goes bad and that you could injure yourself. Make sure you always have a couple flashlights and batteries handy, as you may need them the whole night. Candles also help to have but be careful with those for obvious reasons. (You can get burned or set fire to something!)

With the refrigeration issue, avoid opening the fridge or freezer for as long as possible because it is naturally built to retain its temperature, so by opening and closing it you lose your foods' cold temperature. This can be extended by purchasing a couple bags of ice. It seems stupid but it works way better than you would expect and it's really cheap.

Evacuation Orders.

These occur when a massive life threatening situation has been detected in a metropolitan area. You may receive a local, state or military issued order to retreat to a new location. This could be due to a natural disaster or a military threat. Either way you should definitely retreat, even if you don't know why. There isn't much to say but pack only essentials and leave as soon as you can because the sooner you leave the sooner you are safe. Be careful when driving because some people tend to drive fanatically in a potentially life threatening instance. Usually you will receive the warning in advance to the event but sometimes it can be sudden.

If you have small children, a chronic illness or a disability, you will want to pack an emergency bag and keep it in a hall closet or your car trunk. Ready.gov has great resources for evacuation preparation.

Natural Disasters

Now we get into the stuff that can really be messy. Natural disasters are large weather events that can occur and cause devastating damage to buildings and houses. If a disaster is predicted, you will receive directions on how to stay safe including if an evacuation is ordered.

Hurricanes

There are some of the most devastating events and semi-common. Most places in the US are safe but warmer areas close to the ocean are at high risk. Hurricanes come with intense rain and lightning, flooding and waves. Sometimes a hurricane's effect is barely noticeable at first but your town or city is still in danger of a hurricane. If you think you are ok because the rain lightens up, you are in the eye of the storm and it will get worse again until the predicted hurricane end occurs. Waves can leave the ocean and be as tall as a building. Flooding can make streets and walkways unsafe to be on. Only an inch of water on a street can lift your car off the ground and turn it into a boat. You do not want to be in a building because of the risk that you may get trapped. The structural integrity of your building will be vastly weakened by the water.

It is best to evacuate the area as all public services are often be eliminated during the storm surges.

Earthquakes

Believe it or not, these tectonic disturbances occur all the time, but they are usually too weak for us to notice. In the event that a larger earthquake strikes, here are a couple tips on how to survive.

In an earthquake, the tremors will shake, knock things off tables, and bring down furniture. Public health researchers studied where people were located when they were found alive days after a deadly event. They discovered that people who lay on the floor NEXT to, not under, large pieces of furniture often survived. The call this area the triangle of life. The floor, the original piece of furniture(often a bed or couch) and a piece of furniture or wall that fell and was caught by the bed, created a triangular space that provided protection and air for someone trapped there. When the wall crashes and hits the original piece of furniture, it often breaks the legs of the furniture crushing anyone under the furniture but creating a triangle of life right next to the sofa or bed.

Tornadoes

Tornadoes are large "wind funnels" that occur in nature. They whip up near-by objects in an intensely powered vacuum. Tornadoes cause large objects including cars, heavy furniture and large posts to come loose and move in unpredictable directions. If you are inside a car, leave as soon as possible because tornadoes can tip cars over. Instead if you are outside, get down on the ground as low as possible, especially in a ditch.   If you are inside go to the basement or lowest level in the house and inside a closet or other area nowhere near a window. Try to leave the area and get as far as possible because tornadoes can easily pull humans into its vortex or hit someone with an object caught in it's whirlwind.

Wildfires

Wildfires are large fires that keep spreading, leaving the area scarred scorched and incinerated. You will usually receive a warning or evacuation order if a wildfire is heading towards your area because usually they start in large forests during the dry season. The best thing to do is pack your car with valuables and necessities and leave the area as soon as possible. If you forgot something and the fire is near your home DO NOT GO BACK AS YOU WILL DIE. Not only will the fire be dangerously close, but the ash emitted will make breathing extremely difficult. You will be better off leaving the area as soon as possible.

Winter Weather

Last thing to be wary of is a snow emergency or heavy snowstorm. These are very dangerous because sometimes they can disable electricity and block people in houses. Also the heavy snow can cave in roofs. Snow emergences are a great example of why you will want a stash of preserved foods and water ready. A generator will also help but isn't necessary. You will have to sit and wait if the snow has reached a dangerously high level because attempting to leave will leave you frozen from the temperatures.

Winter weather can be most dangerous for people who are driving. Roads are slippery and the white lines that show you were to drive disappear in the snow. Sudden gusts of wind can bring so much snow that you suddenly can't see in front of you. In areas where there are lots of roads from point a to point b, driving in a snowstorm often requires slow driving and patience. But in some mountain areas like in the Rocky

Mountains, a snowstorm can stop traffic for hours or days. Having a full tank of gas, extra food, water and warm blankets can save your life. Stay as warm as possible and wait for help because there isn't much else you can do.

Our Story

On July 8, 2019, Karen Laing, a public health educator and health literacy expert sat at the Underground Railroad History Project of the Capital Region and explained to the teens of Albany's summer jobs program, that her group would be writing a health literacy book. They would use her book The Health Literacy Guide for Teens and Young Adults as a starting point, but would have free range to write their own book. Three young men took the challenge.

Ian took on the translation of Karen's book into teen speak. Brandon and Qudratullah (Lucky) did additional research and added their own life experiences into the book. Together the boys finished the book a day earlier than the deadline.

Funding from this book will help to continue to fund the Young Abolitionist's Teen Scholars' Institute at the Underground Railroad Project. Each youth in the program received a copy of the book as well our local school and public libraries. We hope this book will help millions of teens begin to take control of their health and their medical care.

Ian's Story:

I grew up in Albany and have always lived here with my 2 adopted siblings and both my parents. I'm kind of a school hopper going from Mt Moriah to Loudonville Christian to NSES to K.I.P.P. and finally to becoming homeschooled. I signed up for the summer youth employment program looking to buy a new phone with some cash, but what I got was more than that. I found confidence, practical skills, social skills but most importantly, I found out how stupid difficult it is to not curse in a book and also to get up every morning. Life is tough but as you live it you will find different Easter eggs and tricks on how to optimize your life. As long as you have something to look forward too, you will be fine.

Qudratullah's Story:

My whole name Qudratullah Zadran Haidari and I am from Afghanistan in Afghanistan I am from Khost and we have spend a lot of time on this book. I choose this topic because I play a lot of sports and I know people who don't. They are the same age as me but their weight is very high so that's why I choose this topic. I hope this book that I write can change a lot of people's lives. If they do what my group said in the book and I think they will know a lot of stuff by now and I hope you guys do better with everything we said.

Brandon's Story:

Top of the mornin' to ya ladies. My Name is Brandon. Writing this wasn't as easy as you may think. I had to spend so much time researching. While it is fun, it's also quite difficult because there are so many potential websites you can get reliable information from. Also, a lot of what I wrote was pretty hard to write because it's not at all easy to share your own stories about your life. This has easily been one of the most challenging tasks I've done yet. It's also one of the funnest. Hope you all have a lovely day.

www.ingramcontent.com/pod-product-compliance
Lightning Source LLC
Chambersburg PA
CBHW051400280526
45784CB00007B/3034